THE BODY BUILDERS KITCHEN

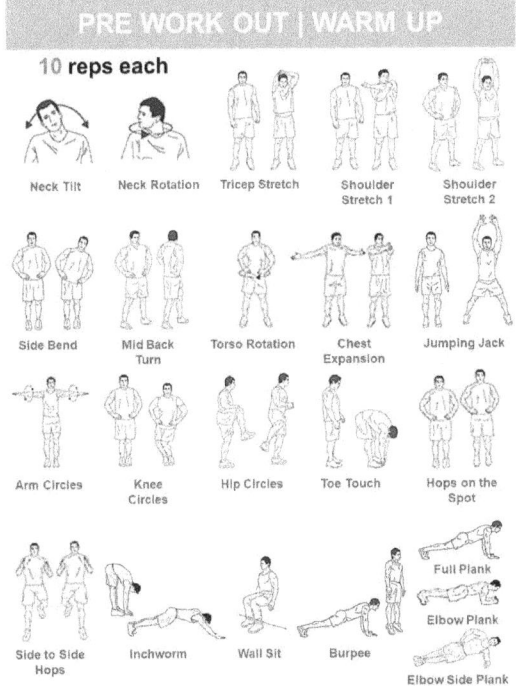

"150 Muscle-building, fat burning recipes with meal plans and workout guide to make you stronger"

GET ACCESS TO MORE BOOKS FROM SAME AUTHOR

ACKNOWLEDGMENTS

This book arose as a collective masterpiece, stitched together by strands of inspiration, commitment, and shared enthusiasm. As I approach the threshold of thankfulness, I feel obligated to express my heartfelt gratitude to those whose influence and support have impacted my creative journey.

Thank you, my muse, for the elusive spark that sparked the creative flames within me. Your gentle whispers danced on the boundaries of my mind, coaxing me to write this story.

A heartfelt thank you to my loved ones, friends, and mentors for patiently listening to my ramblings, providing crucial insights, and offering unfailing encouragement. Your conviction in my talents drove my desire to complete this job.

To the unsung heroes behind the scenes: editors, proofreaders, and cover designers, your diligent labor has turned this text into a polished treasure. Your dedication to perfection has not gone unnoticed, and I am grateful for your knowledge.

Thank you to the literary community, both local and distant, for creating an environment of creation, exchange, and fellowship. The shared experiences and insights have expanded my grasp of the trade, giving this book more substance.

Last but not least, my readers are the heartbeat of this story. Your curiosity and open-mindedness are the wind under my wings. May the pages that follow inspire you, inspiring new ideas and igniting your creativity.

This book demonstrates the power of teamwork and the connection of our experiences. Together, we created something absolutely unique, for which I am eternally thankful.

With deepest gratitude.

[SOPHIA MEGAN]

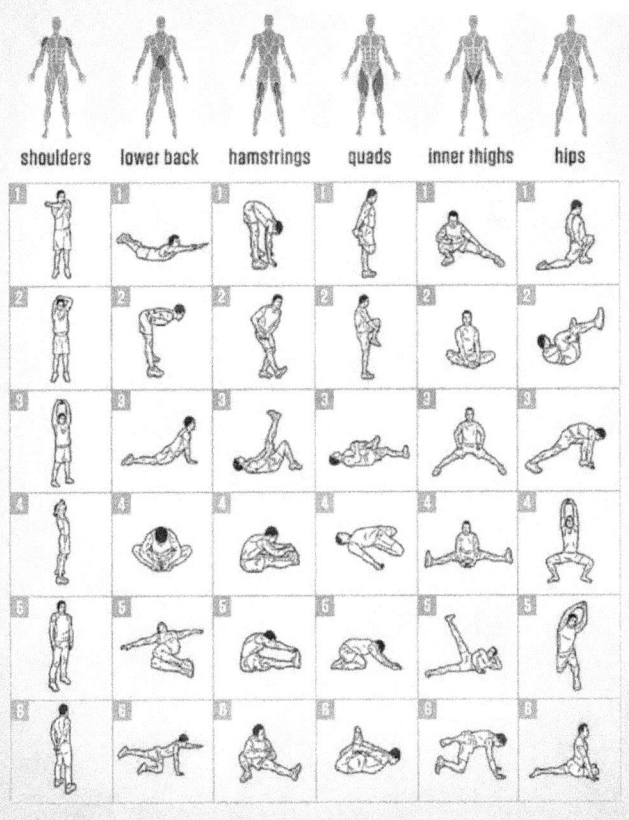

TABLE OF CONTENTS

CHAPTER 3
BREAKFASTS TO FUEL YOUR DAY

Greek yogurt with mixed berries and chopped nuts.

Oatmeal topped with sliced bananas and almond butter.

Protein pancakes with cottage cheese and fruit.

Veggie omelette with whole wheat toast.

Quinoa breakfast bowl with avocado and poached eggs.

High-protein smoothie with whey protein, almond milk, and fruit.

Cottage cheese and pineapple on whole grain toast.

Whole grain cereal with milk and sliced almonds

Sweet potato hash with lean ground turkey.

Chapter 4
PROTEIN-PACKED LUNCHES

Grilled chicken breast with quinoa and steamed broccoli.

Tuna salad with mixed greens, hard-boiled eggs, and avocado.

Turkey and spinach wrap with hummus in a whole wheat tortilla.

Baked salmon with sweet potato and asparagus.

Lentil and chickpea salad with feta cheese and a vinaigrette dressing.

Chapter 5
ENERGIZING SNACKS

Chapter 6
MUSCLE-BUILDING DINNERS
Grilled chicken breast with broccoli and quinoa.

Baked salmon with sweet potato and asparagus.

Lean beef stir-fry with mixed vegetables and brown rice.

Turkey and black bean chili with a side of avocado

Tofu and vegetable curry with brown rice

Pork tenderloin with roasted Brussels sprouts
and mashed cauliflower.

Chapter 7
HYDRATION AND RECOVERY DRINKS
Importance of Hydration for Exercise
Post-Workout Protein Smoothies

Chapter 8
THE WORKOUT GUIDE

Chapter 9:
WEEKLY WORKOUT PLANS
Beginner's 4-Week Workout Schedule

Intermediate Split Routine

Appendix A
Grocery Shopping List
- Essential Foods for Muscle Building
Sample Grocery List

INTRODUCTION

Welcome to The Body Builder's Cookbook

Welcome to The Body Builder's Cookbook, a culinary resource created especially to aid in your quest for physical fitness by offering a delicious selection of filling and savory recipes. This cookbook is your go-to source for cooking meals that not only satisfy your body's nutritional needs but also entice your taste buds, whether you're an experienced bodybuilder, an aspiring fitness enthusiast, or simply someone trying to adopt a better lifestyle.

In the fitness industry, we comprehend that accomplishing your goals calls for more than just going to the gym; it's about developing a holistic approach that includes both exercise and eating. In order to maximize performance, promote muscle growth, and speed up recovery, proper nutrition is essential. But who said wholesome cuisine had to be bland and uninteresting journey.

So, whether you're flipping through these pages for inspiration, seeking to revamp your meal plan, or embarking on a brand-new fitness adventure, The Body Builder's Cookbook is your culinary partner. Get ready to embark on a flavorful expedition that marries your love for food with your dedication to a healthier, fitter you. Your body is a temple, and the food you nourish it with should be nothing short of extraordinary. Let's dive in and savor the journey of nourishment, growth, and transformation – one delectable bite at a time.

How Nutrition and Exercise Work Together

The relationship between nutrition and exercise is crucial when it comes to achieving your fitness goals and maintaining a healthy lifestyle. Proper nutrition provides the fuel your body needs to perform optimally during exercise and helps in recovery afterward. Let's delve into how nutrition and exercise work together:

- **Energy Balance**: To build a strong and healthy body, you need to strike the right balance between the calories you consume and the calories you expend through physical activity. This balance is known as energy balance. If you consume more calories than you burn, you'll likely gain weight. If you burn more calories than you consume, you'll likely lose weight.

- **Macronutrients**: The three main macronutrients are carbohydrates, proteins, and fats. Each plays a unique role in supporting your body during exercise and recovery.

- **Carbohydrates**: These are your body's primary source of energy, especially during intense workouts. Carbohydrates are stored as glycogen in your muscles and liver, and they provide the quick energy needed for high-intensity exercises.

- **Proteins**: Protein is essential for repairing and building muscle tissues. Engaging in regular exercise increases your protein requirements, as the muscles undergo stress and damage during workouts. Consuming an adequate amount of protein helps in muscle recovery and growth.

- **Fats**: Healthy fats are important for overall health, hormone production, and energy. While they are not the primary source of exercise energy, they become more important during longer, endurance-based activities.

- **Hydration**: Staying properly hydrated is vital for performance and recovery. Water is involved in almost every bodily function, including transporting nutrients, regulating body temperature, and removing waste products. Dehydration can lead to decreased exercise performance and even impair recovery.

- **Pre-Workout Nutrition**: Fueling your body before a workout is essential for sustaining energy levels and preventing muscle breakdown. A balanced meal containing carbohydrates and proteins about 1-2 hours before exercise can provide the necessary nutrients for optimal performance.

- **Post-Workout Nutrition:** After exercising, your body is in a prime state to absorb nutrients. Consuming a meal rich in carbohydrates and protein within the first hour after exercise can help replenish glycogen stores and support muscle recovery.

- **Nutrient Timing**: Timing your meals around your workout schedule can enhance your results. For example, consuming carbohydrates before a high-intensity workout can provide energy, while consuming protein after your workout can aid in muscle repair.

- **Supplements**: While whole foods should be your primary source of nutrients, supplements can be used to fill in nutritional gaps. Common supplements include protein powder, creatine, BCAAs (branched-chain amino acids), and vitamins/minerals.

- **Individualization**: Everyone's nutritional needs are different based on factors such as age, gender, body composition, activity level, and fitness goals. It's important to tailor your nutrition plan to your specific needs.

CHAPTER ONE

BUILDING THE BODY FOUNDATION

Understanding Your Body's Nutritional Needs

Before you embark on your journey towards building a stronger and fitter body, it's crucial to have a solid understanding of your body's nutritional needs. Proper nutrition forms the foundation upon which your fitness goals are built. This section will delve into the key macronutrients and micronutrients that play a vital role in supporting muscle building, optimizing performance, and maintaining overall well-being

Key Macronutrients for MuscleBuilding

- **Protein**: Often hailed as the cornerstone of muscle building, protein is made up of amino acids, the building blocks of muscle tissue. Including an adequate amount of protein in your diet supports muscle repair and growth, especially after intense workouts. Sources of high-quality protein include lean meats, poultry, fish, eggs, dairy products, legumes, tofu, and plant-based protein powders.

- **Carbohydrates**: Carbohydrates are your body's primary source of energy. They fuel your workouts and aid in replenishing glycogen stores in muscles. Complex carbohydrates, like whole grains, fruits, vegetables, and legumes, provide sustained energy and are preferable over simple sugars.

- **Fats**: Healthy fats are essential for hormone production, cell structure, and overall health. They also contribute to energy reserves, especially during low-intensity activities. Opt for sources such as avocados, nuts, seeds, olive oil, fatty fish, and coconut oil.

Micronutrients for Optimal   Performance

While macronutrients provide the energy and building blocks, micronutrients are equally important for various physiological processes that support your fitness journey:

- *Vitamins*: These organic compounds are essential for various bodily functions, including energy metabolism, immune system support, and antioxidant protection. Vitamins like vitamin C (found in citrus fruits), vitamin A (abundant in leafy greens), and the B vitamins (found in whole grains and lean meats) are crucial for overall health and performance.

- **Minerals**: Minerals play roles in bone health, muscle contraction, fluid balance, and more. Key minerals for fitness include calcium (found in dairy products), magnesium (found in nuts and seeds), and iron (found in lean meats and legumes).

- *Electrolytes*: Sodium, potassium, chloride, and other electrolytes help maintain proper fluid balance, nerve function, and muscle contractions. These are especially important during intense workouts to prevent dehydration and cramping.

- **Antioxidants**: Found in colorful fruits and vegetables, antioxidants help combat oxidative stress caused by intense exercise. They contribute to recovery and overall health by reducing inflammation and cell damage.

CHAPTER TWO

DESIGNING YOUR MEAL PLAN

Designing a meal plan for a bodybuilder requires careful consideration of their caloric intake goals, meal timing for energy and recovery, as well as pre-workout and post-workout nutrition. Here's a comprehensive guide to help you create an effective meal plan:

Setting Your Caloric Intake Goals

The first step is to determine your daily caloric needs. This will depend on factors such as your age, gender, weight, height, activity level, and goals (bulking, cutting, or maintaining). Generally, bodybuilders aiming to build muscle often need a caloric surplus, while those cutting want a deficit.

Meal Timing for Energy and Recovery

Spacing out your meals throughout the day can help maintain steady energy levels and support muscle recovery. Consider the following meal timing strategy:

- **Breakfast**: Kickstart your day with a balanced meal containing complex carbohydrates (oats, whole grains), lean protein (eggs, Greek yogurt), and healthy fats (avocado, nuts).

- **Mid-Morning Snack**: Opt for a protein-rich snack like a protein shake, cottage cheese, or a handful of nuts.

- **Lunch**: Prioritize lean protein sources (chicken, turkey, tofu), complex carbs (brown rice, quinoa), and plenty of vegetables.

- **Afternoon Snack**: Choose a combination of protein and carbs, such as a whole grain wrap with turkey and veggies.

- **Dinner**: Similar to lunch, include lean protein, complex carbs, and veggies. Consider adding fatty fish (salmon, mackerel) for omega-3 fatty acids.

- **Evening Snack**: A casein protein shake, Greek yogurt, or a small portion of nuts can provide sustained protein release overnight.

Pre-Workout and Post-Workout Nutrition

Pre-Workout and Post-Workout Nutrition:
Proper pre-workout and post-workout nutrition is crucial for optimizing performance and recovery.

- **Pre-Workout**: Consume a balanced meal 1-2 hours before exercise. Include easily digestible carbs (fruit, white rice) for quick energy, and lean protein (chicken, fish) to support muscle preservation during the workout. Avoid heavy fats and fiber that might cause digestive discomfort.

- **Intra-Workout**: For longer, intense workouts, consider a carbohydrate-electrolyte drink to maintain energy levels.

- **Post-Workout**: Consume a meal rich in both protein and carbs within 1-2 hours after your workout. This helps replenish glycogen stores and supports muscle recovery. A whey protein shake with a banana or a turkey sandwich on whole grain bread are good options.

CHAPTER 3

BREAKFASTS TO FUEL YOUR DAY

These breakfast samples will help you have an energy-filled day..

Scrambled eggs with spinach and turkey bacon.

Ingredients:
Eggs
Spinach
Turkey bacon
Salt and pepper to taste

Instructions:
- Cook the turkey bacon in a skillet until crispy. Remove and set aside.
- In the same skillet, add the spinach and sauté until wilted. Remove and set aside.
- In a bowl, whisk the eggs and season with salt and pepper.

- Pour the eggs into the skillet and cook over medium heat, stirring gently until they're scrambled to your desired consistency.
- Mix in the cooked spinach and crumbled turkey bacon. Serve hot.

Greek yogurt with mixed berries and chopped nuts.

Ingredients:
Greek yogurt
Mixed berries (such as strawberries, blueberries, raspberries)
Chopped nuts (such as almonds, walnuts)

Instructions:
- Spoon Greek yogurt into a bowl.
- Top with mixed berries and chopped nuts.
- Enjoy as is or drizzle with honey for extra sweetness.

Oatmeal topped with sliced bananas and almond butter.

Ingredients:
Oatmeal
Bananas
Almond butter

Instructions:
- Prepare oatmeal according to package instructions.
- Slice bananas and place them on top of the oatmeal.
- Drizzle almond butter over the bananas.
- Stir and enjoy.

Protein pancakes with cottage cheese and fruit.

Ingredients:
Pancake mix (can be protein pancake mix)
Cottage cheese
Mixed fruit (such as berries, sliced peaches)

Instructions:
- Prepare the pancake mix according to package instructions.
- Fold the cottage cheese into the pancake batter.
- Cook pancakes on a griddle or skillet.
- Top with mixed fruit.

Veggie omelette with whole wheat toast.

Ingredients:
- Eggs
- Assorted vegetables (such as bell peppers, onions, tomatoes, spinach)
- Salt and pepper to taste
- Whole wheat toast

Instructions:
- Chop the vegetables.
- In a bowl, whisk the eggs and season with salt and pepper.
- In a skillet, sauté the vegetables until they're cooked.
- Pour the eggs over the vegetables and cook until set.
- Fold the omelet in half and serve with whole wheat toast.

Quinoa breakfast bowl with avocado and poached eggs.

Ingredients:
Quinoa
Avocado
Eggs
Salt and pepper to taste

Instructions:
- Cook quinoa according to package instructions.
- Poach the eggs.
- Slice the avocado.
- In a bowl, layer cooked quinoa, sliced avocado, and poached eggs.
- Season with salt and pepper.

High-protein smoothie with whey protein, almond milk, and fruit.

Ingredients:
Whey protein powder
Almond milk
Mixed fruit
Optional: honey or sweetener of your choice

Instructions:
- In a blender, combine whey protein powder, almond milk, mixed fruit, and sweetener if desired.
- Blend until smooth and creamy. Adjust almond milk for desired consistency.

Cottage cheese and pineapple on whole grain toast.

Ingredients:

Cottage cheese
Pineapple chunks
Whole grain toast

Instructions:

- Spread cottage cheese on whole grain toast.
- Top with pineapple chunks.

Whole grain cereal with milk and sliced almonds.

Ingredients:

- Whole grain cereal
- Milk (dairy or plant-based)
- Sliced almonds

Instructions:
- Pour whole grain cereal into a bowl.
- Add milk.
- Sprinkle sliced almonds on top.

Sweet potato hash with lean ground turkey.

Ingredients:

Sweet potatoes
Lean ground turkey
Onion
Bell peppers
Salt, pepper, and spices of choice

Instructions:

- Dice sweet potatoes, onion, and bell peppers.
- In a skillet, cook lean ground turkey until browned. Remove from skillet.
- In the same skillet, add a little oil and sauté the sweet potatoes, onion, and bell peppers until cooked and slightly crispy.
- Add cooked ground turkey back to the skillet and mix.
- Season with salt, pepper, and desired spices.

Breakfast burrito with scrambled eggs, black beans, and salsa.

Ingredients:
Tortillas (flour or whole wheat)
Eggs
Black beans (canned or cooked)
Salsa
Salt and pepper to taste
Optional toppings: shredded cheese, chopped cilantro, sour cream

Instructions:
- Scramble the eggs in a pan over medium heat until fully cooked. Season with salt and pepper.
- Warm the tortillas in a dry pan or microwave for a few seconds to make them pliable.
- Place a portion of scrambled eggs and black beans on each tortilla.
- Top with salsa and any optional toppings you prefer.
- Fold in the sides of the tortilla and roll it up tightly to form a burrito.

Tofu and vegetable stir-fry with brown rice.

Ingredients:

1. Firm tofu, cubed
2. Mixed vegetables (bell peppers, broccoli, carrots, snap peas, etc.)

3. Cooked brown rice
4. Soy sauce
5. Sesame oil
6. Garlic and ginger (minced)
7. Salt and pepper to taste
8. Optional toppings: chopped green onions, sesame seeds

Instructions:
- Heat a tablespoon of sesame oil in a large pan or wok over medium-high heat.
- Add minced garlic and ginger, sauté for a minute until fragrant.
- Add the cubed tofu and stir-fry until it's slightly browned on all sides.
- Add the mixed vegetables and continue to stir-fry until they're tender-crisp.
- Season with soy sauce, salt, and pepper.
- Serve the tofu and vegetable stir-fry over cooked brown rice.
- Garnish with optional toppings before serving.

Peanut butter and banana sandwich on whole wheat bread.

Ingredients:
Whole wheat bread slices
Peanut butter
Banana, sliced

Instructions:

- Spread peanut butter on one side of each bread slice.
- Place banana slices on one of the peanut butter-coated bread slices.
- Press the two slices of bread together to form a sandwich.

Smoked salmon on whole grain bagel with cream cheese.

Ingredients:
Whole grain bagel, sliced and toasted
Smoked salmon
Cream cheese
Red onion, thinly sliced
Capers (optional)

Instructions:
- Spread cream cheese on both halves of the toasted bagel.
- Place smoked salmon on one half of the bagel.
- Top with thinly sliced red onion and capers, if using.
- Close the bagel with the other half.

Protein-rich frittata with asparagus and chicken sausage.

Ingredients:
- 6 large eggs
- 1/2 cup cooked chicken sausage, diced

- 1/2 cup asparagus, trimmed and chopped
- 1/4 cup grated cheese (cheddar, mozzarella, or your choice)
- 1/4 cup milk
- Salt and pepper to taste
- 1 tablespoon olive oil

Instructions:
- Preheat the oven to 375°F (190°C).
- In a bowl, whisk together eggs, milk, grated cheese, salt, and pepper.
- Heat an oven-safe skillet with olive oil over medium heat.
- Add the diced chicken sausage and chopped asparagus to the skillet. Sauté for a few minutes until the asparagus is tender.
- Pour the egg mixture into the skillet, distributing it evenly.
- Let the frittata cook on the stovetop for a couple of minutes until the edges start to set.
- Transfer the skillet to the preheated oven and bake for about 15-20 minutes, or until the frittata is cooked through and slightly golden on top.
- Remove from the oven, let it cool slightly, then slice and serve.

Whole grain waffles with low-fat ricotta and berries.

Ingredients:

1 cup whole grain waffle mix (follow package instructions for additional ingredients)
1/2 cup low-fat ricotta cheese
Assorted berries (strawberries, blueberries, raspberries)

Instructions:
- Prepare the whole grain waffle batter according to the package instructions.
- Preheat your waffle iron and lightly grease it.
- Pour the batter onto the waffle iron and cook until the waffles are golden and crispy.
- Spread a dollop of low-fat ricotta cheese on each waffle.
- Top with fresh assorted berries.
- Serve the waffles with ricotta and berries on top.

Chia seed pudding with protein powder and mixed fruit.

Ingredients:
1/4 cup chia seeds
1 cup milk (dairy or plant-based)
1 scoop protein powder (flavor of your choice)
Mixed fruits (such as berries, kiwi, mango), chopped
Honey or maple syrup for sweetness (optional)

Instructions:
- In a bowl, mix chia seeds, milk, and protein powder. Stir well.

- Cover the bowl and refrigerate for at least 2 hours or overnight, allowing the chia seeds to absorb the liquid and create a pudding-like texture.
- Stir the chia seed mixture to ensure even consistency.
- Layer the chia seed pudding and mixed fruits in serving glasses or bowls.
- Drizzle with honey or maple syrup if desired.
- Enjoy the chia seed pudding with protein powder and mixed fruit.

Steak and eggs with sautéed spinach.

Ingredients:
1 steak (such as sirloin or ribeye)
2 eggs
2 cups fresh spinach
Salt and pepper to taste
Olive oil for cooking

Instructions:
- Season the steak with salt and pepper on both sides.
- Heat a skillet or pan over medium-high heat and add a drizzle of olive oil.
- Cook the steak to your desired doneness, flipping once. Cooking times vary depending on the thickness of the steak and your preference.
- While the steak is cooking, in another pan, sauté the fresh spinach with a bit of olive oil until wilted. Season with salt and pepper.

- In a separate pan, cook the eggs (fried, scrambled, or poached) according to your preference.
- Once everything is cooked, plate the steak alongside the sautéed spinach and eggs.
- Season with additional salt and pepper if needed.
- Serve the steak and eggs with sautéed spinach.

Overnight oats with protein powder and grated coconut.

Ingredients:
1/2 cup rolled oats
1 cup milk (dairy or plant-based)
1 scoop protein powder (flavor of your choice)
2 tablespoons grated coconut
Honey or maple syrup for sweetness (optional)
Fresh fruit for topping (bananas, berries, etc.)

Instructions:

- In a container or jar, combine rolled oats, milk, and protein powder. Stir well.
- Add grated coconut and mix.
- If desired, sweeten with honey or maple syrup and stir again.
- Cover the container and refrigerate overnight.
- In the morning, give the oats a good stir.
- Top with fresh fruit before serving.

Turkey sausage with scrambled egg whites and whole grain toast.

Ingredients:
2 turkey sausage links
4 egg whites
Salt and pepper to taste
2 slices whole grain bread, toasted

Instructions:
- Cook the turkey sausage links according to the package instructions (usually in a skillet or oven).
- While the sausages are cooking, whisk the egg whites in a bowl. Season with a pinch of salt and pepper.
- In a non-stick skillet over medium heat, cook the scrambled egg whites, stirring gently until cooked through.
- Toast the slices of whole grain bread.
- Once everything is cooked, plate the turkey sausages, scrambled egg whites, and whole grain toast.
- Enjoy the turkey sausage with scrambled egg whites and whole grain toast.

Chapter 4
Protein-Packed Lunches

Grilled chicken breast with quinoa and steamed broccoli.

Ingredients:

2 boneless, skinless chicken breasts
1 cup quinoa
2 cups water or chicken broth
2 cups broccoli florets
Olive oil
Salt and pepper to taste

Instructions:
- Preheat the grill to medium-high heat.
- Season the chicken breasts with olive oil, salt, and pepper.
- Grill the chicken for 6-8 minutes per side or until fully cooked.
- While the chicken is grilling, rinse the quinoa and cook it according to the package instructions.
- Steam the broccoli until tender, about 5 minutes.
- Serve the grilled chicken over cooked quinoa with steamed broccoli on the side.

Tuna salad with mixed greens, hard-boiled eggs, and avocado.

Ingredients:
2 cans of tuna, drained
4 cups mixed greens
2 hard-boiled eggs, sliced
1 avocado, sliced
Olive oil and vinegar for dressing

Instructions:
- In a large bowl, combine the drained tuna, mixed greens, hard-boiled egg slices, and avocado.
- Drizzle with olive oil and vinegar for dressing. Toss to combine.

Turkey and spinach wrap with hummus in a whole wheat tortilla.

Ingredients:

2 whole wheat tortillas
8 slices of turkey
1 cup fresh spinach leaves
4 tablespoons hummus
Instructions:

- Lay out the tortillas and spread 2 tablespoons of hummus on each.
- Place 4 slices of turkey on each tortilla.
- Top with fresh spinach leaves.
- Roll up the tortillas tightly and cut in half

.

Baked salmon with sweet potato and asparagus.

Ingredients:

2 salmon fillets
2 sweet potatoes, peeled and cubed
1 bunch asparagus spears
Olive oil
Salt and pepper to taste
Instructions:

- Preheat the oven to 400°F (200°C).
- Place the salmon fillets on a baking sheet lined with parchment paper.
- Toss the sweet potato cubes and asparagus with olive oil, salt, and pepper.
- Arrange the sweet potatoes and asparagus around the salmon on the baking sheet.
- Bake for 15-20 minutes or until the salmon flakes easily with a fork and the sweet potatoes are tender.

Lentil and chickpea salad with feta cheese and a vinaigrette dressing.

Ingredients:

1 cup cooked lentils
1 cup cooked chickpeas
1/2 cup crumbled feta cheese
1/4 cup olive oil
2 tablespoons red wine vinegar
1 teaspoon Dijon mustard
Salt and pepper to taste
Instructions:

- In a large bowl, combine the cooked lentils, chickpeas, and crumbled feta cheese.
- In a separate bowl, whisk together the olive oil, red wine vinegar, Dijon mustard, salt, and pepper to make the vinaigrette.
- Drizzle the vinaigrette over the salad and toss to combine.

Beef stir-fry with mixed vegetables and brown rice.

Ingredients:

1 pound beef sirloin, thinly sliced
3 cups mixed vegetables (bell peppers, broccoli, carrots, etc.), sliced
2 cups cooked brown rice
2 tablespoons soy sauce
1 tablespoon sesame oil
1 teaspoon minced garlic
Salt and pepper to taste
Instructions:

In a wok or large skillet, heat the sesame oil over high heat.
Add the sliced beef and minced garlic. Stir-fry until the beef is browned.
Add the mixed vegetables and stir-fry until they are tender-crisp.
Stir in the cooked brown rice and soy sauce. Season with salt and pepper.

Cook for an additional 2-3 minutes, stirring constantly, until everything is heated through

Greek yogurt parfait with berries, nuts, and honey.

Ingredients:

1 cup Greek yogurt
1/2 cup mixed berries (strawberries, blueberries, raspberries)
2 tablespoons mixed nuts (almonds, walnuts), chopped
1 tablespoon honey
Instructions:

In a glass or bowl, layer Greek yogurt, mixed berries, and chopped nuts.
Drizzle honey over the top.

Cottage cheese and pineapple bowl with mixed nuts.

Ingredients:

1 cup cottage cheese
1/2 cup pineapple chunks
2 tablespoons mixed nuts (cashews, pistachios), chopped
Instructions:

In a bowl, combine cottage cheese and pineapple chunks.
Sprinkle chopped mixed nuts on top.

Egg white omelette with spinach, tomatoes, and low-fat cheese.

Ingredients:

4 egg whites
Handful of fresh spinach
1/2 cup diced tomatoes
1/4 cup low-fat shredded cheese
Salt and pepper to taste
Instructions:

In a bowl, whisk the egg whites with salt and pepper.
In a non-stick skillet, sauté the spinach and diced tomatoes until wilted.
Pour the egg whites over the vegetables and cook until set.
Sprinkle shredded cheese on one half of the omelette, fold it in half, and cook for another minute until the cheese is melted.

Black bean and quinoa bowl with salsa and diced chicken.

Ingredients:

1 cup cooked quinoa
1 cup black beans, drained and rinsed
1/2 cup salsa
1 cup cooked diced chicken breast
Fresh cilantro, chopped (optional)
Instructions:

In a bowl, combine cooked quinoa, black beans, salsa, and diced chicken.

Garnish with chopped fresh cilantro if desired.

Roast beef and Swiss cheese sandwich on whole grain bread.

Ingredients:
- 8 slices whole grain bread
- 1/2 pound roast beef, thinly sliced
- 4 slices Swiss cheese
- Mustard or mayo (optional)
- Lettuce and tomato slices

Instructions:
- Lay out the slices of bread and spread mustard or mayo if desired.
- Layer the roast beef, Swiss cheese, lettuce, and tomato slices on 4 slices of bread.
- Top with the remaining bread slices to make sandwiches.

Shrimp and avocado salad with mixed greens and a citrus dressing.

Ingredients:
- 1/2 pound shrimp, cooked and peeled
- 2 avocados, sliced
- 4 cups mixed greens
- Citrus dressing (orange juice, lemon juice, olive oil)
- Salt and pepper to taste

Instructions:

- In a large bowl, combine the cooked shrimp, sliced avocados, and mixed greens.
- Drizzle with the citrus dressing and season with salt and pepper.
- Toss gently to combine.

Tofu and vegetable stir-fry with sesame seeds and brown rice.

Ingredients:
- 1 block firm tofu, cubed
- Assorted stir-fry vegetables (bell peppers, broccoli, snap peas, etc.)
- 2 cups cooked brown rice
- 2 tablespoons soy sauce
- 1 tablespoon sesame seeds
- Sesame oil
- Minced ginger and garlic

Instructions:
- In a wok or large skillet, heat sesame oil and sauté minced ginger and garlic.
- Add the cubed tofu and stir-fry until lightly browned.
- Add the stir-fry vegetables and cook until tender.
- Stir in the cooked brown rice, soy sauce, and sesame seeds.
- Cook for a few more minutes until heated through.

Roasted turkey and vegetable quinoa bowl.

Ingredients:
- 1 cup cooked quinoa
- 1/2 pound roasted turkey, sliced
- Assorted roasted vegetables (zucchini, bell peppers, carrots, etc.)
- Olive oil
- Herbs of choice (rosemary, thyme)
- Salt and pepper to taste

Instructions:
- In a bowl, combine cooked quinoa, sliced roasted turkey, and roasted vegetables.
- Drizzle with olive oil, sprinkle with herbs, salt, and pepper. Toss gently.

Greek salad with grilled chicken, olives, and feta cheese.

Ingredients:
- 2 boneless, skinless chicken breasts, grilled and sliced
- Mixed salad greens
- Kalamata olives
- Crumbled feta cheese
- Cucumber slices, red onion slices
- Greek dressing

Instructions:
- In a bowl, combine mixed salad greens, cucumber slices, and red onion slices.

- Top with grilled chicken, Kalamata olives, and crumbled feta cheese.
- Drizzle with Greek dressing.

Smoked salmon and cream cheese whole wheat wrap.

Ingredients:
- 2 whole wheat tortillas
- 4 ounces smoked salmon
- 2 tablespoons cream cheese
- Thinly sliced red onion, capers
- Fresh dill

Instructions:
- Lay out the tortillas and spread cream cheese on each.
- Place smoked salmon on top, followed by red onion, capers, and fresh dill.
- Roll up the tortillas tightly and cut in half.

Chickpea and spinach curry with basmati rice.

Ingredients:
2 cups cooked chickpeas
2 cups fresh spinach
Curry sauce (coconut milk, curry paste, spices)
Cooked basmati rice

Instructions:
- In a pan, heat the curry sauce and add cooked chickpeas.

- Once heated, add fresh spinach and cook until wilted.
- Serve the chickpea and spinach curry over cooked basmati rice.

Grilled lean steak with roasted Brussels sprouts and mashed sweet potatoes.

Ingredients:

- Lean steak
- Brussels sprouts, halved
- Sweet potatoes, peeled and diced
- Olive oil
- Salt and pepper to taste

Instructions:

- Grill the lean steak to your desired doneness.
- Toss Brussels sprouts in olive oil, salt, and pepper. Roast in the oven.
- Boil sweet potatoes until tender, then mash with a bit of olive oil, salt, and pepper.
- Serve the grilled steak with roasted Brussels sprouts and mashed sweet potatoes

Chicken and black bean burrito bowl with salsa and guacamole.

Ingredients:

- Grilled chicken, sliced
- 1 cup cooked black beans
- 1 cup cooked rice
- Salsa
- Guacamole

- Optional toppings: shredded cheese, sour cream, chopped cilantro

Instructions:
- In a bowl, layer cooked rice, black beans, and sliced grilled chicken.
- Top with salsa and guacamole.
- Add any optional toppings you prefer.

Mixed bean salad with diced turkey and a balsamic vinaigrette.

Ingredients:
- Mixed beans (kidney beans, black beans, etc.), cooked and drained
- 1/2 pound cooked turkey, diced
- Chopped vegetables (bell peppers, red onion, etc.)
- Balsamic vinaigrette
- Fresh herbs (parsley, basil)

Instructions:
- In a bowl, combine mixed beans, diced turkey, and chopped vegetables.
- Drizzle with balsamic vinaigrette and sprinkle with fresh herbs.

Chapter 5
ENERGIZING SNACKS

Snacks play a crucial role in a bodybuilder's diet as they help provide the necessary nutrients and energy to fuel workouts, support muscle growth, and aid in recovery. When selecting snacks for bodybuilding, it's essential to prioritize options that offer a balance of protein, carbohydrates, healthy fats, and micronutrients. Here are some ideal snack choices for bodybuilders:

- *Protein Bars*: Protein bars are convenient and come in various flavors. Look for bars with at least 20 grams of high-quality protein, minimal added sugars, and a decent amount of fiber. They provide a quick source of protein for muscle repair and growth.

- *Greek Yogurt*: Greek yogurt is rich in protein, low in sugar, and contains probiotics that promote gut health. It's a great choice to support muscle recovery and overall well-being. You can add fruits, nuts, or honey for added flavor and nutrients.

- *Nut Butter with Whole Grain Bread or Rice Cakes*: Nut butters like almond, peanut, or cashew are packed with healthy fats and protein. Pair them with whole grain bread or rice cakes for a balanced snack that provides sustained energy.

- **Cottage Cheese:** Cottage cheese is high in protein and low in fat. It's a versatile option that can be combined with fruits, vegetables, or nuts to enhance taste and nutritional value.

- **Hard-Boiled Eggs:** Eggs are a fantastic source of complete protein, vitamins, and minerals. Hard-boiled eggs are portable and can be seasoned with salt, pepper, or your preferred spices for added flavor.

- **Trail Mix**: Make your trail mix by combining nuts, seeds, dried fruits, and a touch of dark chocolate. This snack provides healthy fats, protein, and carbohydrates for energy and satiety.

- **Hummus with Veggies**: Hummus is a protein-rich dip made from chickpeas. Pair it with carrot sticks, cucumber, celery, or bell pepper slices for a nutrient-dense and satisfying snack.

- **Tuna or Salmon Packets**: Pre-packaged tuna or salmon packets are a convenient source of lean protein. They're easy to carry and can be eaten straight from the pouch or combined with whole-grain crackers.

- **Low-Fat String Cheese**: String cheese is a convenient, portable snack that's high in protein and calcium. It's a quick and easy way to support muscle health.

- ***Fruit Smoothies:*** Blend fruits like bananas, berries, and spinach with protein powder, Greek yogurt, and almond milk for a delicious an

CHAPTER 6
MUSCLE-BUILDING DINNERS

Muscle-building dinners play a crucial role in the development and maintenance of lean muscle mass, which is essential for overall health and fitness. These dinners are carefully planned to provide the body with the necessary nutrients to support muscle growth, repair, and recovery, especially after intense workouts. Here are few dinner you should test as a body builder:

Grilled chicken breast with broccoli and quinoa.
Ingredients:

- 2 boneless, skinless chicken breasts
- 1 cup quinoa
- 2 cups water or chicken broth
- 2 cups broccoli florets
- Olive oil
- Salt and pepper, to taste
- Lemon wedges (optional, for garnish)

Instructions:
- Preheat your grill to medium-high heat.
- Season the chicken breasts with salt, pepper, and a drizzle of olive oil.
- Grill the chicken for about 6-8 minutes per side or until cooked through.
- While the chicken is grilling, rinse the quinoa under cold water and cook it according to the package instructions using water or chicken broth.
- Steam the broccoli until tender, about 4-5 minutes.
- Serve the grilled chicken on a plate with quinoa and steamed broccoli. Garnish with lemon wedges if desired.

Baked salmon with sweet potato and asparagus.

Ingredients:

- 2 salmon fillets
- 2 sweet potatoes, peeled and diced
- 1 bunch asparagus, trimmed
- Olive oil
- Salt and pepper, to taste
- Lemon slices (optional, for garnish)

Instructions:

- Preheat your oven to 375°F (190°C).
- Place the sweet potato cubes and trimmed asparagus on a baking sheet.
- Drizzle with olive oil, sprinkle with salt and pepper, and toss to coat.
- Place the salmon fillets on the same baking sheet.
- Season the salmon with salt, pepper, and a drizzle of olive oil.
- Bake in the preheated oven for 15-20 minutes, or until the salmon flakes easily with a fork and the sweet potatoes are tender.
- Garnish with lemon slices if desired and serve.

Lean beef stir-fry with mixed vegetables and brown rice.

Ingredients:

- 1 lb lean beef, thinly sliced

- 2 cups mixed vegetables (bell peppers, broccoli, carrots, snap peas, etc.)
- 2 cups cooked brown rice
- 2 tablespoons low-sodium soy sauce
- 1 tablespoon vegetable oil
- 1 clove garlic, minced
- 1 teaspoon ginger, minced
- Salt and pepper, to taste

Instructions:

- In a large skillet or wok, heat the vegetable oil over high heat.
- Add the minced garlic and ginger, and sauté for about 30 seconds.
- Add the sliced beef and stir-fry until it's no longer pink. Remove the beef from the skillet and set it aside.
- Add the mixed vegetables to the skillet and stir-fry for 3-5 minutes until they are tender-crisp.
- Return the cooked beef to the skillet, add soy sauce, and stir to combine.
- Season with salt and pepper to taste.
- Serve the beef and vegetable stir-fry over cooked brown rice.

Turkey and black bean chili with a side of avocado.

Ingredients:

- 1 lb ground turkey
- 1 can (15 oz) black beans, drained and rinsed

- 1 can (14.5 oz) diced tomatoes
- 1 onion, chopped
- 1 bell pepper, chopped
- 2 cloves garlic, minced
- 1 tablespoon chili powder
- 1 teaspoon cumin
- 1 teaspoon paprika
- Salt and pepper, to taste
- Avocado slices (for garnish)
- Sour cream (optional, for garnish)
- Shredded cheese (optional, for garnish)

Instructions:

- In a large pot or Dutch oven, heat olive oil over medium heat. Add chopped onions and bell peppers and sauté until they become tender, about 5 minutes.
- Add the minced garlic and cook for an additional minute.
- Add the ground turkey and cook until it's no longer pink, breaking it apart with a spoon as it cooks.
- Stir in the chili powder, cumin, paprika, salt, and pepper.
- Add the black beans and diced tomatoes to the pot, and bring the mixture to a simmer.
- Reduce the heat to low, cover, and let the chili simmer for about 20-30 minutes, stirring occasionally.

- Serve the turkey and black bean chili with avocado slices and optional garnishes like sour cream and shredded cheese.

Tofu and vegetable curry with brown rice.
Ingredients:

- 1 block (14 oz) tofu, cubed
- 2 cups mixed vegetables (bell peppers, broccoli, carrots, snap peas, etc.)
- 1 can (14 oz) coconut milk
- 2 tablespoons curry paste (red or green, depending on your preference)
- 1 tablespoon vegetable oil
- 1 onion, chopped
- 2 cloves garlic, minced
- 1 tablespoon ginger, minced
- Salt and pepper, to taste
- Cooked brown rice, for serving

Instructions:
- Heat vegetable oil in a large skillet or wok over medium-high heat.
- Add chopped onion and sauté until it becomes translucent.
- Stir in the minced garlic and ginger and cook for another minute.
- Add the cubed tofu and stir-fry until it's lightly browned on all sides.
- Mix in the curry paste and cook for 1-2 minutes until fragrant.

- Pour in the coconut milk and bring the mixture to a simmer.
- Add the mixed vegetables and simmer for about 10-15 minutes or until the vegetables are tender.
- Season with salt and pepper to taste.
- Serve the tofu and vegetable curry over cooked brown rice.

Pork tenderloin with roasted Brussels sprouts and mashed cauliflower.

Ingredients:

- 1 pork tenderloin (about 1 lb)
- 1 lb Brussels sprouts, trimmed and halved
- 1 head cauliflower, cut into florets
- Olive oil
- Salt and pepper, to taste
- 2 cloves garlic, minced
- 1/4 cup milk (or milk alternative)
- Butter (or butter alternative, optional)
- Fresh herbs for garnish (e.g., parsley or thyme)

Instructions:

- Preheat your oven to 400°F (200°C).
- Place the trimmed and halved Brussels sprouts on a baking sheet, drizzle with olive oil, season with salt and pepper, and toss to coat. Roast for about 20-25 minutes, or until they are tender and slightly browned.

- While the Brussels sprouts are roasting, rub the pork tenderloin with olive oil, minced garlic, salt, and pepper.
- In a separate ovenproof skillet, heat some olive oil over medium-high heat. Sear the pork tenderloin on all sides until it's browned.
- Transfer the skillet with the seared pork to the preheated oven and roast for about 20-25 minutes, or until the internal temperature reaches 145°F (63°C).
- While the pork is roasting, steam the cauliflower florets until they are tender.
- Mash the steamed cauliflower with a potato masher or blend it in a food processor. Add milk and butter (if desired) to reach your preferred consistency. Season with salt and pepper.
- Once the pork is done, let it rest for a few minutes before slicing.
- Serve the sliced pork tenderloin with roasted Brussels sprouts and mashed cauliflower. Garnish with fresh herbs.

Shrimp and spinach salad with quinoa and a vinaigrette dressing.

Ingredients:

- 1 lb large shrimp, peeled and deveined
- 6 cups fresh spinach leaves
- 1 cup cooked quinoa
- 1/4 cup cherry tomatoes, halved
- 1/4 cup red onion, thinly sliced

- 1/4 cup feta cheese (optional, for garnish)
- Olive oil
- Salt and pepper, to taste

For the Vinaigrette Dressing:

3 tablespoons olive oil
1 tablespoon balsamic vinegar
1 teaspoon Dijon mustard
1 clove garlic, minced
Salt and pepper, to taste

Instructions:

- Season the shrimp with salt, pepper, and a drizzle of olive oil.
- Heat a skillet over medium-high heat and cook the shrimp for about 2-3 minutes per side or until they turn pink and opaque. Remove from heat and set aside.
- In a large salad bowl, combine the fresh spinach leaves, cooked quinoa, cherry tomatoes, and sliced red onion.
- To make the vinaigrette dressing, whisk together olive oil, balsamic vinegar, Dijon mustard, minced garlic, salt, and pepper in a small bowl.
- Drizzle the vinaigrette dressing over the salad and toss to coat.
- Divide the salad onto plates and top with the cooked shrimp.
- Garnish with feta cheese if desired.

Grilled steak with sautéed mushrooms and a side of green beans.

Ingredients:

- 2 steak cuts (e.g., ribeye or sirloin)
- 8 oz mushrooms, sliced
- 1 lb fresh green beans, trimmed
- Olive oil
- Salt and pepper, to taste
- Garlic powder (optional)
- Fresh thyme or rosemary (for garnish)

Instructions:

- Preheat your grill to medium-high heat.
- Season the steak cuts with salt, pepper, and a drizzle of olive oil.
- Grill the steaks for about 4-5 minutes per side for medium-rare, or adjust the cooking time to your preferred doneness.
- While the steaks are grilling, heat some olive oil in a skillet over medium heat.
- Add the sliced mushrooms and sauté until they are browned and tender, about 5-7 minutes.
- In a separate pot, steam the trimmed green beans until they are crisp-tender, about 4-5 minutes.
- Season the green beans with salt, pepper, and garlic powder if desired.
- Once the steaks are done, let them rest for a few minutes before slicing.

- Serve the sliced grilled steak with sautéed mushrooms and steamed green beans. Garnish with fresh herbs.

Baked cod with a tomato and basil sauce, served with steamed broccoli.
Ingredients:

- 4 cod fillets
- 1 can (14.5 oz) diced tomatoes
- 1/4 cup fresh basil leaves, chopped
- 2 cloves garlic, minced
- Olive oil
- Salt and pepper, to taste
- 1 lb broccoli florets

Instructions:

- Preheat your oven to 375°F (190°C).
- Place the cod fillets in a baking dish and season them with salt, pepper, and a drizzle of olive oil.
- In a separate bowl, combine the diced tomatoes, chopped fresh basil, minced garlic, salt, and pepper.
- Pour the tomato and basil mixture over the cod fillets.
- Bake in the preheated oven for about 15-20 minutes, or until the cod flakes easily with a fork.
- While the cod is baking, steam the broccoli florets until they are tender, about 4-5 minutes.
- Serve the baked cod with the tomato and basil sauce alongside steamed broccoli.

Lentil soup with a side of mixed greens and a protein source of your choice

Ingredients:

- 1 cup dried green or brown lentils
- 4 cups vegetable broth
- 1 onion, chopped
- 2 carrots, chopped
- 2 celery stalks, chopped
- 2 cloves garlic, minced
- 1 bay leaf
- Salt and pepper, to taste
- Mixed greens (e.g., spinach, arugula, or kale)
- Protein source of your choice (e.g., grilled chicken, tofu, or a hard-boiled egg)

Instructions:

- Rinse the lentils under cold water and drain.
- In a large soup pot, heat some olive oil over medium heat.
- Add the chopped onion, carrots, and celery, and sauté until they become tender, about 5 minutes.
- Add the minced garlic and sauté for another minute.
- Pour in the vegetable broth and add the lentils and bay leaf.
- Bring the mixture to a boil, then reduce the heat to low, cover, and simmer for about 20-25 minutes, or until the lentils are tender.
- Season the lentil soup with salt and pepper to taste.

- Serve the lentil soup with a side of mixed greens and your chosen protein source.

Chapter 7
HYDRATION AND RECOVERY DRINKS

Hydration is a critical aspect of exercise and physical activity, as it plays a fundamental role in maintaining overall health and optimizing athletic performance.

- Importance of Hydration for Exercise

Hydration is crucial for exercise performance and overall health. Staying properly hydrated before, during, and after exercise is essential for several reasons:

- **Optimal Physical Performance**: Dehydration can lead to a significant decrease in physical performance. Even mild dehydration can impair your strength, power, and endurance during exercise, making it harder to achieve your fitness goals.

- **Temperature Regulation**: When you exercise, your body generates heat. Sweat is your body's primary mechanism for dissipating this heat. Dehydration reduces your ability to sweat, which can lead to overheating and an increased risk of heat-related illnesses like heat exhaustion or heat stroke.

- **Energy Levels**: Dehydration can lead to a decrease in blood volume and, consequently, a decrease in blood flow to muscles. This can result in feelings of fatigue and reduced energy levels during exercise.

- **Joint Lubrication**: Proper hydration helps maintain the viscosity of synovial fluid, which lubricates your joints. Inadequate hydration can lead to joint discomfort or stiffness during exercise.

- **Cognitive Function**: Dehydration can impair cognitive function, including focus, concentration, and decision-making. This can be dangerous during exercise, especially in activities that require coordination and precision.

- **Reduced Risk of Injury**: When you're properly hydrated, your muscles and joints are more resilient. Dehydration can increase the risk of muscle cramps, strains, and ligament injuries.

- *Recovery*: After exercise, rehydration is essential for recovery. It helps restore lost fluids and electrolytes, replenish glycogen stores, and repair damaged muscle tissue. Proper hydration post-exercise can reduce soreness and enhance your body's ability to adapt and improve.

- *Electrolyte Balance:* Sweating not only expels water but also important electrolytes like sodium, potassium, and chloride. Maintaining the proper balance of these electrolytes is critical for muscle function, nerve signaling, and overall health.

- Post-Workout Protein Smoothies

After workout it's necessary to regain lost energy. With these simple and easy smoothies, You can get back lost energy and have an energy filled day.

Chocolate Peanut Butter Protein Smoothie

Ingredients:
1 scoop chocolate protein powder
2 tbsp peanut butter
1 banana
1 cup almond milk
Ice cubes (optional)
Instructions:
- Blend all the ingredients until smooth.

Berry Blast Protein Smoothie

Ingredients:
1 cup mixed berries (strawberries, blueberries, raspberries)
1 scoop vanilla protein powder
1/2 cup Greek yogurt
1 cup water or almond milk
Honey or sweetener to taste (optional)
Instructions:
- Combine all ingredients in a blender and blend until well mixed.

Green Power Protein Smoothie

Ingredients:
1 scoop vanilla protein powder
1 cup spinach leaves
1/2 avocado
1/2 banana
1 cup unsweetened coconut water
Instructions:
- Blend all ingredients until smooth.

Mango Pineapple Protein Smoothie

Ingredients:
1 scoop vanilla protein powder
1/2 cup mango chunks
1/2 cup pineapple chunks

1 cup coconut milk
Ice cubes (optional)

Instructions:
- Blend until creamy and smooth.

Almond Joy Protein Smoothie

Ingredients:
1 scoop chocolate protein powder
2 tbsp unsweetened shredded coconut
1 tbsp almond butter
1 banana
1 cup almond milk

Instructions:
Blend all the ingredients until well combined.

Strawberry Banana Protein Smoothie

Ingredients:
1 scoop strawberry protein powder
1 banana
1 cup strawberries
1 cup almond milk
Ice cubes (optional)
Instructions:
Blend until smooth.

Peachy Keen Protein Smoothie

Ingredients:
1 scoop vanilla protein powder
1 cup frozen peach slices
1/2 cup Greek yogurt
1 cup unsweetened almond milk

Instructions:
Blend until creamy and peachy.

Tropical Paradise Protein Smoothie:

Ingredients:
1 scoop vanilla protein powder
1/2 cup pineapple chunks
1/2 cup mango chunks
1/2 banana
1 cup coconut water

Instructions:
Blend until it feels like a tropical vacation in a glass.

Oatmeal Cookie Protein Smoothie:

Ingredients:
1 scoop vanilla protein powder
1/2 cup rolled oats
1/2 tsp cinnamon
1 tbsp almond butter
1 cup unsweetened almond milk

Instructions:

Blend until it tastes like an oatmeal cookie.

Cherry Almond Protein Smoothie:

Ingredients:
1 scoop vanilla protein powder
1 cup frozen cherries
2 tbsp almond butter
1 cup almond milk
Ice cubes (optional)

Instructions:
Blend until creamy and cherrylicious.

Chapter 8

THE WORKOUT GUIDE
- Crafting Your Fitness Plan

- **. Set Clear Goals**: Determine what you want to achieve with your fitness plan. Whether it's building muscle, losing weight, improving endurance, or all of the above, having clear goals will help you stay motivated.

- **. Assess Your Current Fitness Level**: Understand where you currently stand in terms of strength, endurance, and overall fitness. This will help you create a plan tailored to your needs.

- **Create a Schedule**: Decide how many days per week you can commit to working out. Be realistic and choose a schedule that fits your lifestyle.

- **Choose Your Activities**: Select a variety of exercises that align with your goals. This may include strength training, cardiovascular exercises, flexibility training, and more.

- **Progressive Overload**: Gradually increase the intensity, duration, or weight of your exercises over time to challenge your body and continue making progress.

- **Nutrition**: Pay attention to your diet. Proper nutrition is essential for reaching your fitness goals. Consult a dietitian or nutritionist if needed.

- **Rest and Recovery**: Don't forget to incorporate rest days into your plan. Rest is crucial for muscle recovery and overall well-being.

- **Tracking and Evaluation**: Keep a workout journal to track your progress. Periodically evaluate your plan to make necessary adjustments.

Strength Training Techniques

Strength training is a form of exercise focused on increasing your muscle strength and endurance. There are various techniques and principles you can employ to optimize your strength training routine. Here are some key strength training techniques:

- 1. **Progressive Overload**:This is the foundation of strength training. You gradually increase the resistance (weight) or intensity of your workouts over time. This progression challenges your muscles to adapt and grow stronger.

- 2. **Compound Exercises**:Compound exercises work multiple muscle groups simultaneously, making them efficient for building strength. Examples include squats, deadlifts, bench presses, and pull-ups.

- 3. **Isolation Exercises**: While compound exercises are crucial, isolation exercises target specific muscles. Examples include bicep curls, tricep extensions, and calf raises. These can help balance your muscle development.

- 4. **Proper Form**:Maintaining correct form is essential for safety and effectiveness. Poor form can lead to injuries and hinder progress. Consider working with a trainer or using mirrors and video recordings to assess your form.

- 5. **Range of Motion (ROM)**:Perform exercises through their full range of motion. This maximizes muscle activation and flexibility. Avoid using momentum to lift weights; instead, focus on controlled movements.

- 6. **Sets and Repetitions**: Adjust the number of sets and repetitions (reps) based on your goals. For strength, aim for fewer reps (1-6) with heavier weights. For endurance, use lighter weights and higher reps (12+).

- 7. **Rest Between Sets**: Allow sufficient rest between sets to recover. For strength and power, longer rest periods (2-5 minutes) are beneficial. For hypertrophy (muscle growth), shorter rests (30-90 seconds) may be more appropriate.

- 8. **Variety:**Change your exercises and routines regularly to prevent plateaus and keep your workouts engaging. This can involve altering the order of exercises, using different equipment, or trying new movements.

- 9. **<u>Periodization</u>**:This involves structuring your training program into distinct phases, such as strength, hypertrophy, and endurance. Each phase has specific rep and set schemes to optimize your progress.

- 10. **<u>Warm-Up and Cool Down</u>**: Always warm up before lifting heavy weights to increase blood flow and reduce the risk of injury. Cooling down helps your body recover and can include stretching and light cardio.

- 11. **<u>Nutrition</u>**: Proper nutrition is vital for muscle recovery and growth. Ensure you're consuming an adequate amount of protein, carbohydrates, and healthy fats. Stay hydrated and consider supplements if needed.

- 12. **<u>Rest and Recovery:</u>** Muscles need time to repair and grow. Adequate sleep and rest days are crucial. Overtraining can lead to injuries and hinder progress.

- 13. **<u>Tracking Progress</u>**:Keep a workout log to track your progress. This helps you adjust your program as needed and stay motivated as you see improvements.

- 14. **Safety**: Always prioritize safety when strength training. Use appropriate equipment, ask for help when needed, and start with lighter weights to master proper form before progressing to heavier loads.

- 15. **Form and Technique Practice:** Dedicate time to practice and perfect your exercise techniques, especially for complex movements like squats and deadlifts.

- 16. **Flexibility and Mobility**: Incorporate flexibility and mobility exercises into your routine to prevent injuries and improve your range of motion.

- **Recovery Techniques:**Consider using recovery techniques such as foam rolling, stretching, and massage to alleviate muscle soreness and improve overall recovery.

Remember that strength training is a long-term commitment, and results may not be immediate. Be patient, stay consistent, and consult with a fitness professional if you're unsure about your training program or technique.

Chapter 9:
WEEKLY WORKOUT PLANS
- Beginner's 4-Week Workout Schedule

This workout plan is designed for those who are new to exercise and want to build a foundation of fitness.

Weeks 1-2: Full-Body Workouts (3 days per week)

Day 1:
- Squats: 3 sets of 10-12 reps
- Push-ups (or knee push-ups): 3 sets of 8-10 reps
- Plank: 3 sets of 20-30 seconds

Day 2:
- Lunges: 3 sets of 10-12 reps per leg
- Dumbbell Rows (if you have access to dumbbells): 3 sets of 8-10 reps per arm
- Bicycle Crunches: 3 sets of 12-15 reps per side

Day 3:
- Deadlift (if you have access to a barbell or dumbbells): 3 sets of 10-12 reps
- Bench Dips: 3 sets of 8-10 reps
- Superman (back extension): 3 sets of 15-20 seconds

Weeks 3-4: Full-Body Workouts (3 days per week)

Continue with the same exercises but increase the intensity by adding weights or increasing repetitions.

- Intermediate Split Routine

This plan is for individuals who have some experience with working out and are looking to target specific muscle groups on different days.

Day 1: Upper Body
- Bench Press: 4 sets of 8-10 reps
- Pull-ups or Lat Pulldowns: 4 sets of 8-10 reps
- Dumbbell Shoulder Press: 3 sets of 10-12 reps
- Bicep Curls: 3 sets of 10-12 reps
- Tricep Dips: 3 sets of 10-12 reps

Day 2: Lower Body
- Squats: 4 sets of 8-10 reps
- Romanian Deadlifts: 4 sets of 8-10 reps
- Leg Press: 3 sets of 10-12 reps
- Calf Raises: 3 sets of 12-15 reps

Day 3: Rest or Light Cardio

Day 4: Core and Cardio
- Plank: 4 sets of 20-30 seconds
- Russian Twists: 3 sets of 12-15 reps per side

- High-Intensity Interval Training (HIIT) or steady-state cardio for 20-30 minutes

Day 5:
You can incorporate a full-body workout for variety if desired.

Day 7: Rest

Appendix A
Grocery Shopping List
- Essential Foods for Muscle Building
Grocery shopping for muscle building requires a well-balanced selection of foods that provide the necessary nutrients to support your fitness goals. Here's a list of essential foods for muscle building and a sample grocery list to get you started:

Protein Sources:

- _Lean meats (chicken, turkey, lean beef)_
- _Fish (salmon, tuna, tilapia)_
- _Eggs_
- _Greek yogurt_
- _Cottage cheese_
- _Tofu or tempeh (for vegetarians/vegans)_

Carbohydrate Sources:
- _Brown rice_
- _Quinoa_
- _Sweet potatoes_

- *Oats*
- *Whole wheat pasta*
- *Whole-grain bread*

Healthy Fats:
- *Avocado*
- *Nuts (almonds, walnuts, cashews)*
- *Seeds (chia seeds, flaxseeds)*
- *Olive oil or coconut oil*
- *Fatty fish (salmon, mackerel)*

Dairy or Dairy Alternatives:
- *Low-fat milk or plant-based milk (e.g., almond, soy, or oat milk)*
- *Cheese (in moderation)*
- *Low-fat or Greek yogurt (mentioned earlier as a protein source)*

Fruits and Vegetables:
- *Leafy greens (spinach, kale)*
- *Broccoli*
- *Bell peppers*
- *Berries (blueberries, strawberries)*
- *Bananas*
- *Apples*

Legumes:
Chickpeas
Black beans
Lentils

<u>Snacks and Supplements</u>:
Protein powder (whey or plant-based)
Protein bars (with minimal added sugar)
Rice cakes
Trail mix (with nuts and dried fruits)
Nut butter (peanut, almond, or other choices)

<u>Additional Items</u>:
Spices and herbs (for flavor without added calories)
Low-sugar condiments (salsa, mustard)

<u>Hydration</u>:
Water and electrolyte-rich beverages

<u>- Sample Grocery List</u>
Sample Grocery List:
- Chicken breasts or thighs
- Salmon fillets
- Eggs
- Greek yogurt
- Quinoa
- Sweet potatoes
- Whole wheat pasta
- Avocado
- Almonds
- Chia seeds
- Olive oil
- Low-fat milk or almond milk
- Spinach
- Broccoli
- Blueberries

- Black beans
- Chickpeas
- Whey protein powder (or a plant-based alternative)
- Rice cakes
- Spices and herbs of your choice

This is just a basic sample grocery list. You can adjust the quantities and specific items based on your personal preferences and dietary restrictions. Make sure to balance your macronutrients (protein, carbohydrates, and fats) according to your fitness goals and consult with a nutritionist or dietitian if you have specific dietary needs. Additionally, remember to stay hydrated and maintain a well-rounded diet to support muscle building and overall health.